Healing without Medication:

25 Best Alternative Recipes to Stay Healthy Without Pills During the Whole Winter

Table of contents

Introduction

When the first signs of winter hit, you can usually tell because either you or all the people around you start to cough, sneeze and complain of "not feeling well." If you have little ones at home, you really know when the seasons are changing, because sickness becomes just another part of the routine. Germs, coughs, colds, the flu, and everything that comes along with it just seems to get past from one member of the family to another until virtually everyone has been sick.

And just when everyone seems to be feeling better, another string of another virus enters the house and you start another round of pass around the cold. For parents and families the winter season can seem to last forever and there doesn't seem to be a week or month when someone isn't sick fighting something or another.

Sometimes the biggest battle we fight is what to do for our families when they are sick. What medicine do we buy? What daytime, nighttime drugs are out there? What dosage is safe for our kids these days? Is there a new regulation on how much is safe based on age or weight? And if we buy this medicine is it even going to give relief to those that are suffering?

Sometimes we spend money and time in the grocery or drug store trying to find the right medicine or even preventative care items and then they don't even work. It's extremely frustrating when all we're trying to do is take care of ourselves or those we love.

Wouldn't it be nice if there were easier, cheaper and more convenient things we could do to bring relief to those we loved and to ourselves? There is. There are home remedies that will bring relief and the care that you need without all the hassle and stress of pills. You can make them in the comfort of your own home with just a little research.

You can and you will understand just how easy it is to know and understand the difference between relying on the pills and store bought medicines to making bringing your own medicine to your loved ones and even to yourself.

Chapter 1 – Home Remedies in the Kitchen

You'll be amazed at how many great home remedies you probably already have in your kitchen. There are so many things that we have in the kitchen that has great health benefits and healing abilities for us. They also work as health boosters, too. So many of them will help in a preventative way to boost our immune systems. In other words, once you kick your cold you can continue using them to help prevent catching another one! Here are several recipes and important things to keep in your kitchen on a consistent basis during the winter season and how to use them!

1) Garlic – Garlic is one of the strongest home remedies out there. It really can and will take on almost any illness you come across. It is known for it's antibacterial effect in the body; so don't be afraid to get some into the body at the first sign of an illness. If you are feeling brave, give this a shot:

   2 cloves of minced garlic

   4-6 ounces of cold water

   Let the garlic sit in the water for 10-20 seconds and then drink. It won't taste great, so drink it fast.

   Note: If you are pregnant or may be pregnant, you should reduce the garlic to one clove (pregnant women should only consume one clove of garlic per day). Also, if it isn't obvious, kids usually don't do well with this recipe.

2) Garlic (part 2) – Here's another great garlic recipes you can try that will give you the same healing effects, but will taste a whole lot better. You might even be able to sneak some to kids.

½ clove of garlic

½ lemon

1 t honey

8 ounces boiling water

Mince the garlic clove and put it into the bottom of a mug. Squeeze the juice from half a lemon. Add in the water and stir. Then add in the honey to taste. Repeat twice a day for as long as you continue to have symptoms.

3) Cinnamon – Cinnamon is probably more commonly known to help with blood sugar, but it also helps to lower fevers in both children and adults. It also has antibiotic properties to help with the common cold and flu. If you are feeling sick, try the following recipe to make a nice soothing tea. It should help to give relief to coughs and any congestion you might be experiencing.

8 oz. hot water

1 T cinnamon

1 t honey

Stir all three ingredients together until the honey dissolves and the cinnamon mixes in. Drink while still hot for best relief.

4) Kitchen Herbs – There are several kitchen herbs that are great for putting together things for you to use while you are sick. Three herbs you'll want

to have around are thyme, rosemary and oregano. These three herbs will help increase your ability to fight the virus or bacteria by boosting your immune system while also getting rid of any congestion in your lungs. Here is a recipe for a steam bath for your face.

2 C boiling water

1-2 t thyme

1-2 t rosemary

1-2 t oregano

After the water is boiling, add the herbs to the water and take it off the heat. Place a lid over the pot and let it sit for 3-5 minutes. After the time has lapsed, remove the lid and hold your face over the pot to breathe in the steam. If desired, wrap a towel over your face. Continue to breathe the steam from the pot as long as you like – 10-15 minutes or until there is no longer steam coming from the pot.

5) Ginger – Ginger is a great way to help your body fight various illnesses you may catch during the winter season. First of all, it can fight against nausea and vomiting, if you happen to catch the flu. If you catch a cold virus, you can also use ginger to reduce your fever or fight a headache. Here's a great recipe for fresh ginger tea:

Homemade Ginger Tea

1-2 C boiling water

Fresh ginger root

½ fresh lemon (optional)

Place your water on the stove to boil. While it is heating up, cut your ginger root into smaller pieces (not extremely small, about the size of a grape. Once your water starts to boil, add your fresh ginger root to the water and let it steep in the water for about 12-15 minutes. Reduce your heat to a simmer during the 12-15 fifteen minutes.

After 15 minutes, strain out the remaining ginger pieces, add the juice from half a lemon and any sweetener you prefer, but neither is necessary just makes the drink a little more enjoyable.

Add the liquid to a mug and enjoy.

6) Yarrow – Yarrow is extremely helpful to help with the cold and flu during the winter season. It isn't commonly found in stores, but can be found if you have an herbal remedy store in your area or if you grow it yourself and dry the leaves and flowers. It has great medicinal purposes not only for colds and flu, but others as well. If you catch an illness within the first 24 hours of catching it and take yarrow, you usually can shorten the illness by leaps and bounds! Here is a great tea recipe as well using the dried yarrow leaves and flowers.

2 t dried yarrow

16 oz. boiling water

1 t lemon juice

2 t sugar (or your favorite sweetener to taste like honey)

Place the yarrow leaves and flowers into your boiling water and let it steep for 8-10 minutes. If you leave it in for longer it will become too bitter, so remove it promptly after ten minutes. Strain your liquid and add in the lemon juice and chosen sweetener. Add more if desired. Stir to combine and let the sweetener dissolve before consuming. Enjoy while still hot.

7) Chamomile – People tend to love chamomile once they are introduced to it. Chamomile is great for people of all ages, including children. It is most commonly known for helping people sleep, but it can also help to lower fevers and reduce inflammation. Because it has a nice taste to it, kids usually don't mind drinking it, which is helpful for parents. It can be used when kids have a fever both to help them sleep and help to reduce the fever during the night. Here is a great nighttime tea recipe.

4 T chamomile leaves

One sprig mint

8 ounces boiling water

Place the chamomile leaves and mint sprig into a pot or tea infuser and then pour in eight ounces of boiling water. Let the tea steep for four to five minutes. After five minutes, remove the tea leaves and mint sprig. Drink while still hot. Note: Cut the recipe in half for children or reduce the amount of chamomile leaves.

8) Vitamin C – This is one of those well-known vitamins that all of our mothers and father probably told us when we were children, but the truth is that they were right. Vitamin C is probably the best Vitamin out there to help with a fast recovery. However, studies have shown that taking the pill form of vitamin C isn't as effective as getting it the natural way. So consider these top vitamin C rich foods in your diet.

Oranges – who doesn't love a good orange? A large orange will give you over 100% of your daily value of vitamin C. Perfect for when you have a cold and need a little extra.

Strawberries – ½ a cup of strawberries will give you 70% of your daily value of Vitamin C. Not to bad, right? They taste delicious and will get you on the road to recovery.

Broccoli – Okay, I know they aren't everyone's favorite, but there have to be a few people out there that don't hate them. Just a ½ a cup of cooked broccoli will give you over 100% of your daily value. Maybe you can muscle some down to help you get better, right?

Kale – Again, maybe not the top of everyone's list, but this leafy vegetable packs a big Vitamin C punch with one cup giving us 134% of our daily value. Maybe consider making yourself a fruit smoothie and throwing it in?

Red Peppers – Just ½ cup of raw red peppers will give you over 100% of your daily value. If you don't want to eat them plain, maybe consider cooking them with some eggs or throwing them in to make fajitas. Adding them into your diet somewhere is going to give you the vitamins.

9) Dried Kitchen Herbs (part 2) – There are some lesser known kitchen herbs that are great for keeping around and will serve you and your family over and over again through the winter season. We've talked a little about a couple of these in their own categories, because they deserved their own sections, but now let's talk about making a Herbal Tincture that will help both kids and adults. Most people agree that it is better than most medicines you buy over the counter at the store to. It helps with colds and coughs and will help to reduce fevers, too.

1/3 C chamomile flowers (dried)

1/3 C yarrow flowers (dried)

1/3 C peppermint leaf (dried)

1/3 C catnip herb (dried)

high proof vodka*

Place all the ingredients, except the vodka, into a mason jar. Pour your vodka over the top of the mason jar filling it ½ to 2/3 full, but making sure all the herbs are covered (this depends on the size of mason jar you use). Let the mixture steep in the jar for two weeks, but it will do better if you let it steep for two months. Shake it everyday while it is steeping.

After two months, use a cheesecloth or small strainer to strain the liquid from the herbs into a new glass jar and the medicine is ready for use. It is safe to use on anyone over the age of two. Give 8-10 drops as needed.

*100 proof vodka is preferred for this recipe, but it is usually extremely hard to find. I have had success with 80 proof vodka as well, when I couldn't find 100 proof.

10) Apple Cider Vinegar – This is probably something you already have in your cupboard, but may not know about all the amazing uses for it. Apple cider vinegar has truly great healing properties for the body, but it does taste awful. You will rarely find a child that you'll be able to convince to take apple cider vinegar, but if you're sick enough as an adult, you'll probably be able to choke it down, or you can't taste anything anyway.

If you need apple cider vinegar to work for you, the first thing to try is gargling it. Put a tablespoon of apple cider vinegar into eight ounces of water and start gargling it. Unfortunately, you don't get to spit it out, just gargle, then drink, gargle, and then drink. It sounds weird and disgusting, but it does work. Continue to repeat the process every hour until you start to feel better.

The apple cider vinegar works on your system immediately by flushing out the virus or bacteria. You should start to feel better as the apple cider vinegar relieves your worst symptoms.

11) Natural Root Cough Syrup – Okay, this one is a great recipe that needed to be here, but is full of so many great ingredients that not one ingredient could shine over another. There are several ingredients that you'll notice we've already talked about for their own specific sections (cinnamon, ginger, etc.), but there are other great ones in here like licorice root and marshmallow root, too, which help with coughs and sore throats. So essentially this recipe is just a powerhouse of ingredients to help you or your loved ones battle whatever illness may come.

2 T licorice root

2 T marshmallow root

2 T ground cinnamon

2 T ginger (fresh and chopped)

8 C water

2 C honey

In a large saucepan, stir together all the ingredients except the honey over low heat. Stirring occasionally, watch the mixture cook until it has reduced by about half (maybe ten minutes). After this time, use a strainer and take out all the herbs. Pour the remaining liquid back into the saucepan. Turn your heat down to the lowest setting and add in your honey. Let it continue to cook for 10-12 minutes.

After 10 minutes, remove it from the heat and pour it into a glass jar (like a mason jar) with a tight lid. It is ready for immediate use. Store in the refrigerator for up to four weeks. You can take 1-2 T, three times a day to relieve a cough, sore throat or any type of congestion.

Chapter 2 – Home Remedies using Essential Oils

Essential oils are also an effective way to fight the illnesses that are so common this time of year. Essential oils may appear somewhat expensive at first sight, but when you realize just how far a bottle of essential oils can go, you'll realize that you only use a small amount each time you make a remedy. One bottle of oil can last you an entire winter season, sometimes two. So the investment into essential oils is one that will pay you back tenfold when you consider the money you'll save in other over the counter medicines you would have bought instead.

Let me say one quick note about essential oils. You do get what you pay for with essential oils. You can buy them cheap online or in big commercial stores, but you'll soon learn the hard way (I did), that you don't have a nice product. When a recipe tells you to add five drops, you'll have to add ten in order to get the same effect. You'll have to decide if paying for a cheaper product is worth it in the longer run.

12) Oregano Oil – Oregano oil is great to help the body fight both viruses and bacteria that you may come across during the winter. It has power as an antibiotic and antiviral oil. You can use it in a diffuser when you first feel signs of sickness. Since oregano doesn't smell the best in your diffuser, you can also rub a few drops on your feet diluted with a carrier oil before going to sleep at night and you'll feel relieved symptoms in the morning.

13) Thyme Oil – You can use thyme oil in a similar fashion to oregano oil however it is not recommended for diffusers. If you choose to rub it on your skin, always use a carrier oil as well. You can even use kitchen olive oil as a carrier oil. Thyme helps to fight off various types of infections in the body. Note: if you are pregnant or may become pregnant, you should not use thyme oil. Younger children should also not use thyme oil, as it will irritate their skin.

14) Peppermint Oil – Peppermint oil is great for this time of year. Come on who doesn't love the smell of peppermint in the winter? It will help to fight viruses and also helps as an antiseptic as well. The best way to use peppermint oil is with your diffuser. Place a few drops in your diffuser and enjoy the smell through the house. They even make humidifiers now with small trays for oils that act as a diffuser.

15) Tea Tree Oil – Tea tree oil is also known as Melaleuca, so don't be confused when you are purchasing oils and can't find one or the other. They are essentially the same thing. This is a powerhouse oil and will help you fight a virus or bacteria. It also can help as an antiseptic, too. It can be rubbed on the skin diluted with a carrier oil to help fight congestion. However because it's such a powerhouse, one of the best ways to use it is as a prevention! Here's a great recipe for a tea tree oil hand sanitizer.

30 drops Tea Tree oil

10 drops Lavender oil

10 drops Clove oil

1 T witch hazel

8 oz. aloe vera gel

Get a medium size glass bowl and place all your essential oils together, let them blend for thirty seconds to a minute. Then add in your aloe vera and witch hazel. Stir these together and make sure everything is well blended. Transfer everything to a jar with a lid and store out of the sunlight in a dark place for four weeks. It is ready for use immediately, but needs to be stored out of the sunlight while using.

Note: Because it doesn't have the same alcohol content as the stuff you buy at the store, it won't keep as long. If you want to make a smaller amount, cut the recipe in half, so you don't end up wasting any.

16) Eucalyptus Oil - Eucalyptus oil is a great way to relieve coughs and colds. Direct application of Eucalyptus oil will relieve your cough. Make a rub with a carrier oil (like olive oil) and then apply to your chest or your throat to bring instant relief from coughs or congestion. The smell alone will help to clear your sinuses and you can repeat as often as needed.

17) Lavender Oil – Lavender is a great oil for fighting viruses in your home. It also helps with sleep. You'll see many products with lavender to help babies and adults fall asleep faster. However, lavender can also help fight colds and flu during the winter season by helping with congestion. Here is a great recipe that combines the use of Lavender and Eucalyptus.

12 drops Eucalyptus oil

8 drops Lavender

2 travel sized tissue packages

Using a dropper, take the tissues and place half the Eucalyptus and half the lavender drops on each opened package of tissue packages. Try and spread out the oils onto different places and different tissues as much as possible while still keeping them folded. Then let them dry. Put them in new Ziploc bags for later use. Use as needed to help relieve congestion.

18) Lemon Oil – Lemon oil is great if you are experiencing a cough or cold. It can also help to relieve congestion. If you are fighting any of these things, take a dropper or your finger and rub the lemon oil directly onto your skin. It will relieve congestion, so rub it on your throat or chest to give you relief from congestion or coughing.

19) Cinnamon Bark – Cinnamon bark is a great way to fight viruses in the house. Again, you can use a diffuser to help fight the viruses by simply pumping the oils into the air. Here is a great recipe for using cinnamon bark and few other oils.

5 drops Cinnamon bark oil

5 drops Clove oil

5 drops Lavender oil

5 drops Sweet Orange oil

Take all of your oils and blend them together in a small glass bottle (preferably dark). After the oils have blended together, use a dropper to place a few drops at a time into a diffuser. Enjoy the smell and the fact that you are fighting the viruses around you!

20) Rosemary Oil – Rosemary is a less common oil, but a great one for winter illnesses. It helps to relieve symptoms connected with both colds and the flu because it acts as both an antiseptic and also as an antimicrobial agent. There is a great recipe that will put together a few oils including Rosemary to help with congestion and headaches associated with winter illnesses.

3 drops Rosemary oil

2 drops Lemon oil

2 drops Eucalyptus oil

In a small bowl or dish blend all three oils together and let sit for a minute to ensure they have come together. After a minute use your fingertip to take a small amount of the mixture and massage it into your temples, the bridge of the nose, the cheekbones, or anywhere else you might be feeling congestion.

Chapter 3 – Home Remedies Found Around the House

Sometimes the traditional things that mom always taught you or maybe the things you heard from grandma are the ways that will give you the most relief. Here are some things from around the house (some you may have and some you may need to get) that will help you get relief from those winter ailments!

21) Heat – We've talked about the oils, but often they aren't associated with the heat and the steam. We all love a good hot bath or shower when we aren't feeling good. There is a reason why we love that. Heat is an important part of healing and feeling better. If you are feeling congested or stuffy, steam and heat can really help to open you up and help you feel better. Here is a great recipe (using one of those essential oils), to open you up and improve your breathing. You can switch out the Eucalyptus in this recipe for tea tree, peppermint, lemon, etc. You could also do a combination if you're brave. It really is up to you.

10 drops Eucalyptus oil (less if you might be sensitive)

Boiling Water (4-5 cups)

Towel

Glass Bowl

Use a dropper to put the essential oil(s) in the bottom of a glass bowl and pour several cups of steaming/boiling water in over the top. Place your face as close as is comfortable to the bowl (don't get to close that you burn your face, but try to get as close as you can) and breathe in the steam. Relax and take in some deep breaths. Use the towel to place over your head and face to keep the steam trapped around you.

If you become too warm or light headed at any point, remove the towel and step away from the bowl to take in some fresh air.

It may also help to have some Kleenex around, because you may need to blow your nose! You can repeat this as often as you like, but usually three times during the day is preferable. You can also adjust how much essential oil you want to add to the water, some people like more or less.

22)Coconut Oil – Coconut oil is extremely helpful for many reasons. It's really not an oil, but more of a solid that when melted becomes an oil. Many people keep it around for various reasons – cooking, cleaning and even beauty products. Here is one you many not have thought of before. Use coconut oil to help you feel better. Here is a coconut oil recipe with some essential oils to create a balm to relieve congestion and any coughing.

2 T Coconut oil

16 drops Eucalyptus oil

10 drops Lavender oil

4 drops Thyme oil

Get yourself a nice dark glass jar. Take the coconut oil first and then mix in the essential oils one by one. You'll be thrilled with the results. Remember we talked about all the great uses for each essential oil – Eucalyptus for the congestion or coughing and thyme to help battle your viruses. Lavender will help calm and relax you. What a fabulous combination, and not to mention that it does smell fantastic together.

23)Hydrogen Peroxide – When you first feel like you are getting sick, hydrogen peroxide can help to prevent you from continuing to get sicker. You can put just a couple drops of hydrogen peroxide in your ears to help prevent infection. If you have extremely sensitive skin you may want to forgo on this one. Young kids and children should also be wary of this option as well.

24) DIY Salt Water Rinse – Sometimes you just need to get your nose clear and it doesn't seem to work by just blowing your nose the traditional way. The nice thing is that by doing a rinse, you can clear up your congestion and you can also clear up your congestion, too. It's like clearing out two birds with one stone. You'll feel so much better in the long run. Here's a great recipe to make your on salt water rinse, so you don't have to spend the bucks on those expensive rinses at the store.

3-4 t salt (iodine-free)

1 t baking soda

Mix this all together and place it in a Tupperware. When you are ready to use, take a teaspoon of this mixture and mix it with eight ounces of warm water (preferably distilled).

Then take a bulb syringe and fill it up with the solution and gently squirt it up your nose while leaning over the sink, bathtub or a pot to catch the water as it come back out. While you're squirting up one side, plug the other side of your nose to help relieve the congestion on one side. Then work on the other side.

25) Epsom Salt – Many people love Epsom salt for a variety of reasons. It is so helpful around the house to clean, cook, and rejuvenates the body.

When you are trying to get through a winter illness, look no further than a great Epsom salt bath for a little help! Here is a great recipe using Epsom salt and few essential oils for smell. The essential oils can be traded out or blended differently depending on your preferences.

2 C Epsom salt

6 drops Eucalyptus oil

6 drops Peppermint oil

6 drops Lavender oil

First measure out your Epsom salt in the dish you plan to store everything in. It needs to be a small glass dish or container with a lid. Then in a separate glass bowl or dish, blend together all of your essential oils. Let them blend together for thirty seconds or a minute. Once you feel like they have blended together nicely, add them back to your Epsom salt. Stir the oils and the salt together with a wooden spoon.

When you are ready to take a bath, add just a few tablespoons of the salt/ oil mixture to your bath as the water is filling up in the tub. Enjoy!

Conclusion

When the seasons start to change and fall turns to winter, we want to be excited for the coming holidays and all the festivities. It is hard, however, when we know that with the coming holidays and parties also comes so many germs, viruses and sickness.

When we know that we will be exposed to everything and our kids will come home from school, church and friends' houses with so many different illnesses that it will hard to keep up, we just become overwhelmed. The hard part is that when you go to the store to find over the counter medicines there are so many to choose from and you feel like they all are advertising the same thing.

With these home remedies you can feel prepared for the winter and whatever illnesses, bacteria and viruses might be thrown your way. You can diffuse protections in your home starting today. You can create a hand sanitizer to start protecting your family before the germs even make it into your home. You won't feel unprepared this season because you'll know what to do before those bugs make it into your home.

These home remedies will have your neighbors and friends asking you how your family is so healthy and always healing faster than anyone else in the neighborhood. You'll be so popular and you'll have to ask yourself if you're ready to share your newfound secret with those around you.

FREE Bonus Reminder

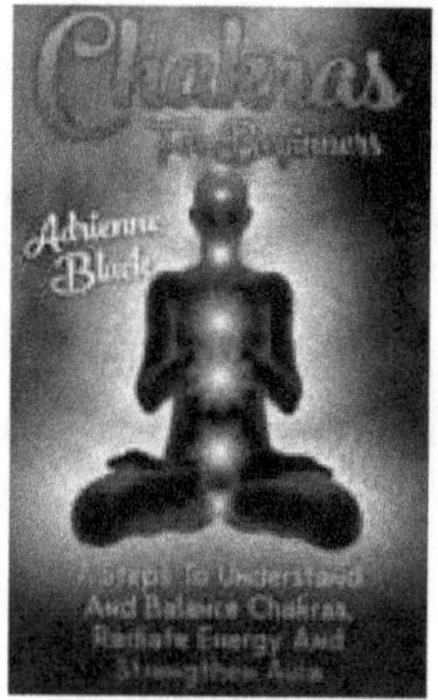

If you have not grabbed it yet, please go ahead and download your special bonus E book *"Chakras for Beginners. 7 Steps To Understand And Balance Chakras, Radiate Energy, And Strengthen Aura"*.

Simply Click the Button Below

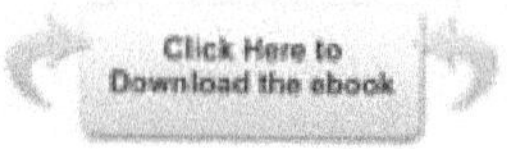

OR Go to This Page

http://lifehacksworld.com/free

BONUS #2: More Free & Discounted Books & Products

Do you want to receive more Free/Discounted Books or Products?

We have a mailing list where we send out our new Books or Products when they go free or with a discount on Amazon. Click on the link below to sign up for Free & Discount Book & Product Promotions.

=> Sign Up for Free & Discount Book & Product Promotions <=

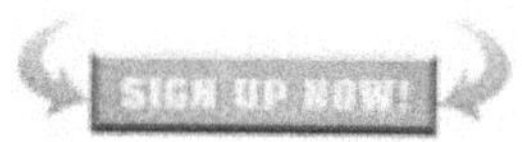

OR Go to this URL

http://zbit.ly/1WBb1Ek

9 781973 829928